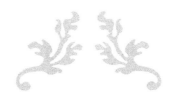

MEDITERRANEAN PIZZA AND BREAD RECIPES

THE BEST RECIPES AND SECRETS TO MASTER THE ART OF ITALIAN PIZZA AND BREAD MAKING

SANDRA RAMOS

MEDITERRANEAN PIZZA AND BREAD RECIPES

_____

_____

_____

_____

SANDRA RAMOS

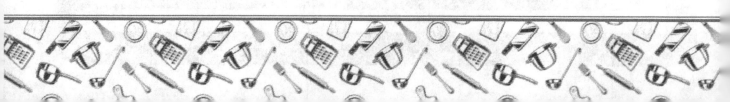

Table of Contents

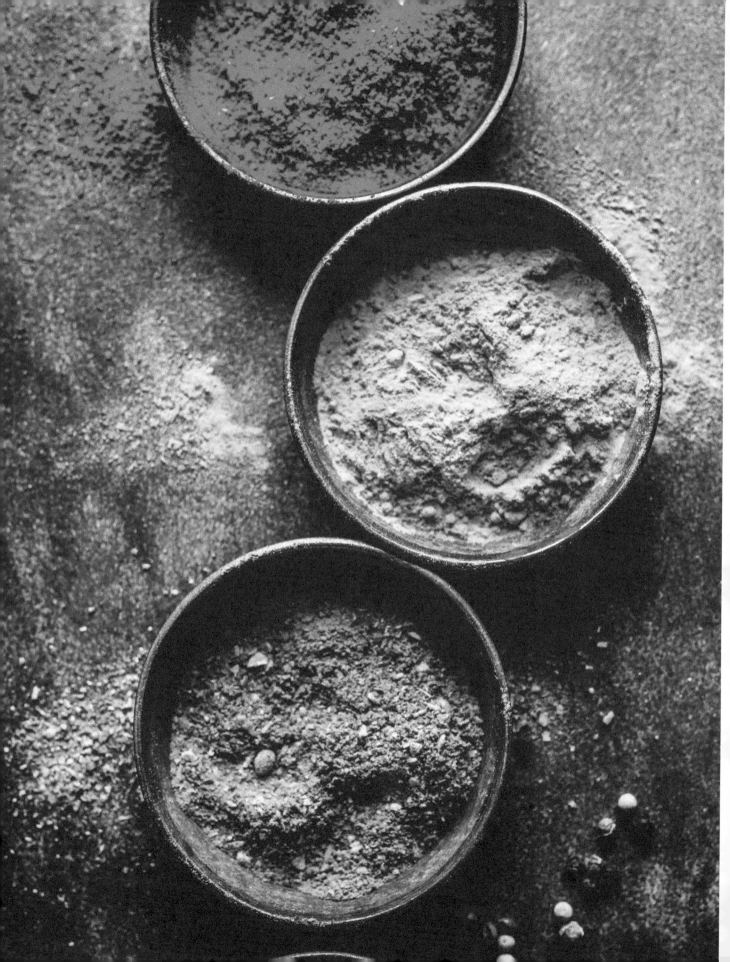

INTRODUCTION

*T**he joy that I am feeling right now cannot be explained. This is because you have chosen me and this book as a guide to a new path – the Mediterranean one. The Mediterranean diet is like no other diet in this world and this way of eating is offering many health and weight benefits.***

Right after World War II, Ancel Keys, a scientist and his colleague Paul Dudley, later known as President Eisenhower's cardiac physician made a Seven Countries Study together with couple of their colleagues. They included people from United States and people from Crete – Mediterranean island. The study was testing these people of all ages and Keys implemented the Mediterranean diet in this study as well.

The 13,000 men came from Netherlands, United States, Greece, Italy, Yugoslavia and Japan and it was estimated that fruits, vegetables, grains, beans and fish are the healthiest ingredients ever. This applies even after considering the impoverishment of WWII. Interestingly this was also estimated at the start, imagine what else they discovered.

Among everything else it was discovered that Mediterranean way of food consumption can make one person lose and maintain healthy weight. Every chapter included in this book will reveal different story about this diet plan and how can you become able to change your eating patterns. Also, you will find out that Mediterranean diet plan gives extreme amount of energy and you will become motivated

Chapter 1: Why this type of diet is the right for you?

Simply because it contains healthy plant foods and it is low in animal foods. Unlike other diets, Mediterranean diet offers more seafood and fish. Seafood and fish are way better than any other meat and the benefits of them is visible after a week or two of constant consumption. Plus, Mediterranean recipes do not leave you hungry, you are full after eating for a longer period.

With constant exercise and fruits, vegetables, legumes, nuts and whole grains (everything that this diet is) you will become the best version of yourself without doubt. Also, you will learn how to perfectly switch bad ingredients with good ingredients. For example, instead of butter you will start using canola or olive oil. Instead of salt you will start using different herbs and spices. Print out the Mediterranean pyramid of foods and you won't regret it.

These recipes are family friendly and you'll be able to host and enjoy and host many gatherings with your friends as well because they are also friend friendly. Occasional glass of red wine is okay, so you are good to go.

HEALTH BENEFITS

Healthy fats are the key component when it comes to Mediterranean cuisine. Also, let's not forget about the most important thing this diet has – plant-based food. Yes, this diet does not remove many food groups, but the mixture of ingredients won't make you a single problem and you will learn what goes with what in time.

But let's elaborate on the health benefits a little bit more. It is scientifically proven that the Mediterranean diet is able to lower the risk of strokes and heart disease. Every patient that has used this diet style so far, has shown lowered levels of oxidized low-density lipoprotein or LDL cholesterol (the bad cholesterol which gets build up in your arteries and causes problems with your heart.

NO MORE HEART PROBLEMS AND STROKES

One of the main ingredients in the Mediterranean diet, extra virgin olive oil, contains alpha-linolenic acid and the Warwick Medical School delivered a study that indicated how olive oil is able to decrease blood pressure. Not only that but also the olive oil is able to lower hypertension because it keeps human arteries clearer and more dilated. Also, it makes the nitric oxide more bioavailable and you won't have problems with cholesterol levels anymore. Only if of course, you consume olive oil (extra virgin) on regular bases.

If you are feeling numbness, weakness, headaches, confusion, vision problems, dizziness or slurred speech do not worry no more. This diet helps and improves this condition together with the ultimate problem – strokes that are happening due to bleeding in the brain or blocked blood vessel.

IMPROVED VISION

Another thing that would improve after starting with this diet is your vision. This diet will help you prevent or stave off the risk of macular degeneration which happens to adults over 54. This disease brings blindness and occurs to over 10 million Americans. Imagine the benefit in here, imagine being victorious against something that is able to destroy your retina and remove the chance of clear vision. The vegetables this diet promotes, the green leafy ones have lutein and that lowers the chance of experiencing cataracts as well.

WEIGHT LOSS

You probably want to lose weight as well and the search for the perfect diet that will be able to provide you that is endless. Until now. This diet is also able to give you the chance to lose weight naturally and easily with nutrient rich foods. The focus in here is on healthy fats while carbohydrates are not that present. They are still here as pasta or bread of course, but their implementation is generally low. The healthy fats, protein and fiber will allow you to lose weight and at the same time will keep you satisfied. Thanks to these nutrients you won't have cravings for candy, chips or cookies no more. The vegetables that you'll consume will fill your stomach and you won't feel hunger for hours. You won't even experience spike in your blood sugar.

IMPROVED AGILITY

According to studies, 70 percent of the seniors who have risk of developing frailty or other muscle weakness lowered the factors of experiencing that by implementing this diet in their lives.

YOU'LL START ENJOYING NATURAL FOODS

This is probably the best thing that this diet brings because it is kind of a new characteristic that you'll develop. As previously noted, this diet is low in sugar and processed foods so its recipes will bring you closer to organic produced foods thus closer to nature. For example, this diet offers honey instead of sugar and this change is priceless.

IMPROVED ASTHMA SYMPTOMS

Another study which included children revealed that antioxidant diet is able to help them decrease their asthma symptoms and at the same time made them not like eating a food that is quite popular – red meat. Yes, this diet helps children to say no to red meat and yes to plant-based food.

NO MORE ALZHEIMER'S RISK

Those people that choose this diet plant without doubt lower their risk of getting Alzheimer's disease in the future. In fact, the latest study shows that getting Alzheimer's is reduced by 40 percent to those people that consume Mediterranean diet foods. Additional exercises are recommended in the process as well.

HELPS PEOPLE WITH DIABETES

Excessive insulin is controlled with Mediterranean diet. Not every diet is able to do this and not every diet can control blood sugar levels and control your weight at the same time. As I told before this diet is at the same time low in sugar and high in healthy acids. This makes a balance for your body and burns fat while gives you energy at the same time.

The American Heart Association reveals that this diet unlike other diets is low in saturated fat while high in fat. This keeps your hunger under control and delivers amazing weight loss results.

MEDITERRANEAN DIET HELPS YOUR BRAIN

Sugar is usually responsible for the highs and lows when it comes to your mood. This diet does not contain artificial sugar at all this your mood and overall brain health will improve as well.

THE WEIGHT LOSS JOURNEY

Planning breakfast, lunch or dinner is not hard, but the part gets tricky when it comes to snacking time. You should make something for yourself that contains from 150 to 200 calories. For example, you can choose apple, pear, grapefruit and a pinch of salt.

The path that this diet offers is the safest when it comes to losing weight. Everything is healthy here and there won't be bouncing.

But many people ask what happens when the time is stumbling on us and when we do not have time to cook the meals present in here. Well, I and this diet of course have a solution for you. Trust me you will like it.

- Fruit slices – pears and apples

- Nut butter – cashew butter, almond butter and more

- Dates and figs

- Tuna salad

- Crackers

- Greek Yogurt

- Olives

- Pitas

- Hummus

Chapter 2: Your Mindset and this diet

In order to remove the unwanted pounds, you have to set your mindset on it like never before. Do not think about that all the time, start thinking about something entirely else while you are focused on losing weight. Or in other words, keep yourself busy while you consume Mediterranean diet foods and you regularly exercise. Also do not expect quick fixes. Time is all you need and after successfully sticking to the plant you'll start to realize the change and how big it is.

To be sincere, the Mediterranean diet is the one thing that you have been missing for so long. You are already motivated I think so all you have to do is start. You already purchased this book, so you are on the right path.

Write down your reasons for starting this journey and every time you are feeling down, or you lack motivated read them out loud. Write down your goals as well. Start with something small and increase as time passes.

Another important thing that people usually forget are their surroundings. It is important for you to surround with people that are positive. Positive mindset regardless of what you do is important, especially when it comes to losing weight and changing something as diet pattern. This is how you'll become able to develop emotionally, healthy realistic goals (do not forget to set your goals first).

Focus on your sleep and develop a healthy sleeping pattern as well. Recharging and sleeping for more than 7 hours are essential when it comes to weight loss because you need extreme amount of energy and sharpness. Good energy and brain sharpness appear only when one is able to properly relax and recharge in the evening hours.

Chapter 3: Nutrition and Portions

Start being aware of the things you consume now. Develop your management skills and stick to the guidelines that this book gives. What to consume? Well start with:

- Vegetables – raw and leafy

- Fruit

- Legumes

- Grains (one slice of bread is allowed)

- Dairy

- Meat

- Potatoes

- Nuts

This is the food you must start combining and portions that include these ingredients will make you set and ready for reaching your goals.

This is a sustainable diet so you won't have serious problems, but I will be lying if I say that cravings won't appear. If you successfully understand your cravings, you'll remove them and soon be proud of your dietary success. Remember, cravings for certain foods indicate need of something entirely else, something that your body is need of.

So, the adjustments that you have to make regarding the cravings are:

- Remove salty cravings with couple of nuts or seeds because your body want silicon.

- Remove fatty and oily foods with spinach, broccoli, cheese and fish because your body wants calcium and chloride.

- Remove sugary foods with chicken, beef, lamb, liver, cheese, cauliflower and broccoli because your body wants phosphorous and tryptophan.

- Remove chocolate cravings (this is the hardest one) with spinach, nuts, seeds, broccoli and cheese because your body wants magnesium and chromium.

You also have to:

- Learn how to recognize every healthy ingredient on the labels. Take back everything that does not look good to your or that indicates that there are many artificial preservatives present.

- Check your serving size.

- Always calculate your calories intake

- Consume food rich in calcium, iron, fiber, vitamin A and vitamin C.

Do not consume:

- Added sugar or foods like candy, soda, ice cream and more.

- Refined oils – soybean oil, canola oil cottonseed oil and more.

- Trans fats – margarine, soda, processed meats, beverages, table sugar and more.

- Processed meat.

- Refined grains.

Foods that you should consume:

- Seafood and Fish: Mussels, clams, crab, prawns, oysters, shrimp, tuna, mackerel, salmon, trout, sardines, anchovies, and more

- Poultry: Turkey, duck, chicken, and more

- Eggs: Duck, quail, and chicken eggs

- Dairy Products: Contain calcium, B12, and Vitamin A: Greek yogurt, regular yogurt, cheese, plus others

- Tubers: Yams, turnips, potatoes, sweet potatoes, etc.

- Vegetables: Another excellent choice for fiber, and antioxidants: Cucumbers, carrots, Brussels sprouts, tomatoes, onions, broccoli, cauliflower, spinach, kale, eggplant, artichokes, fennel, etc.

- Seedsand Nuts: Provide minerals, vitamins, fiber, and protein: Macadamia nuts, cashews, pumpkin seeds, sunflower seeds, hazelnuts, chestnuts, Brazil nuts, walnuts, almonds, pumpkin seeds, sesame, poppy, and more

- Fruits: Excellent choices for vitamin C, antioxidants, and fiber: Peaches, bananas, apples, figs, dates, pears, oranges, strawberries, melons, grapes, etc.

- Spices and Herbs: Cinnamon, garlic, pepper, nutmeg, rosemary, sage, mint, basil, parsley, etc.

- Whole Grains: Whole grain bread and pasta, buckwheat, whole wheat, barley, corn, whole oats, rye, quinoa, bulgur, couscous 18

- Legumes: Provide vitamins, fiber, carbohydrates, and protein: Chickpeas, pulses, beans, lentils, peanuts, peas

- Healthy Fats: Avocado oil, avocados, olive oil, olive oil products and olives

- Beverages: Water and tea

- White meat: Consume them but remove the visible fat and skin

- Red meat: You can consume lamb, pork, and beef in small amounts

- Potatoes: Prepare them with caution but consume them because they are excellent source of potassium, vitamin b, vitamin c and fibers.

- Desserts and sweets: consume cakes, biscuits and sweets in extra small amounts.

There is one thing that you can implement that will make your journey even more beautiful – spices and herbs! Traditional Mediterranean diet is filled with different spices and herbs and each has a different health benefit! Believe it or not herbs and spices are able to do that and that is one of the main reasons why people implement them in their diet. Here are the spices you must include and the benefits they bring:

- Anise – improves digestion, reduces nausea and alleviates cramps.

- Bay leaf – treats migraines.

- Basil – aids digestion and reduces anxiety and stress.

- Black pepper – promotes nutrient absorption and speeds up your metabolism.

- Cayenne pepper – increases metabolism and controls your appetite.

- Sweet and spicy cloves – relive pain, gum and tooth pain. Also, kill bacteria, fungal infections and aid digestive problems.

- Fennel – improves bone health.

- Garlic – improves blood sugar levels and helps you lose weight.

- Ginger – serves as diuretic and increases urine elimination.

- Marjoram – promotes healthy digestion and fights type 2 diabetes.

- Mint – treats nasal congestion, nausea, dizziness and headaches.

- Oregano – treats common cold and reduces infections. It also relieves menstrual pain.

- Parsley – improves your skin, prostate, dental health and blood circulation.

- Rosemary – increases hair growth, reduces stress, inflammation and improves pain.

- Sage – improves your digestion problems.

- Thyme – has antibacterial properties.

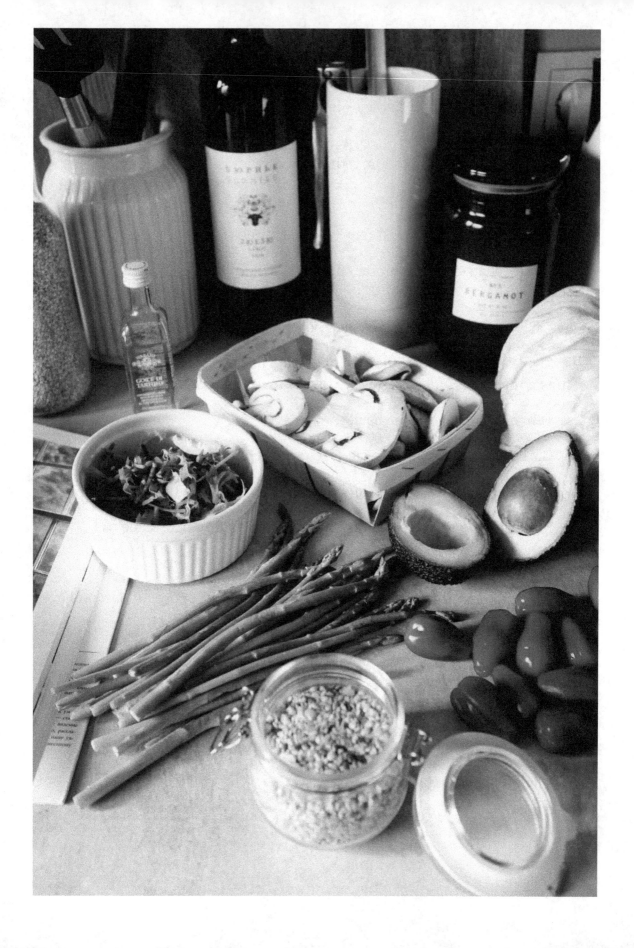

Chapter 4: Exercise

Mediterranean diet is extremely flexible, and you won't have problems while being out with friends. Many recipes in the restaurants come from this particular diet so, you are good to go as long as you do not eat junk food and food that is high in sugar.

Eat slowly and chew your food better. Put your utensils down between bites because that is going to help you slow down the process of eating.

The tips above will help you a lot, but nothing will help you more in this journey than exercising. Two years ago, one scientific research that mainly focused on the Mediterranean diet revealed that this diet is extremely beneficial and gets its full potential when exercise is included. So, to keep your weight under control and to lose weight at the same time you must exercise.

Do not force yourself, start with something easy and small. Spend 30 to 60 minutes daily on that part. Walk, run, do yoga, swim, ride a bike, or simply infiltrate yourself into a regular exercise program online or in a gym near you.

Regular physical activity does not improve only your look, it also improves your strength, mood and balance.

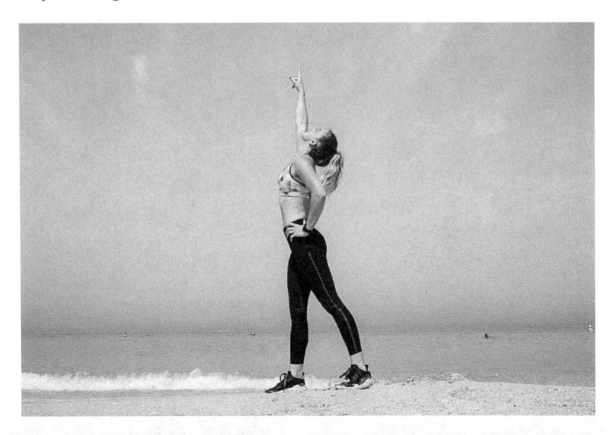

Chapter 5: The recipes in this book

This book contains 500 recipes in total. Each recipe is designed according to the rules Mediterranean diet has. Every recipe is healthy, and every recipe should be made with the best ingredients available – the organic ones. There is also a section for vegans and vegetarians. We wanted to include every person possible in this journey because this journey is all about health and improving yourself and the way you eat. At the bottom of this book you will find a meal plan that we think is going to help you a lot in the few first months. The start won't be that hard, but it is going to be challenging I must admit.

The cooking skills

It is important to know that the Mediterranean do not require hours and hours in the kitchen. The way these recipes are prepared is easy and convenient.

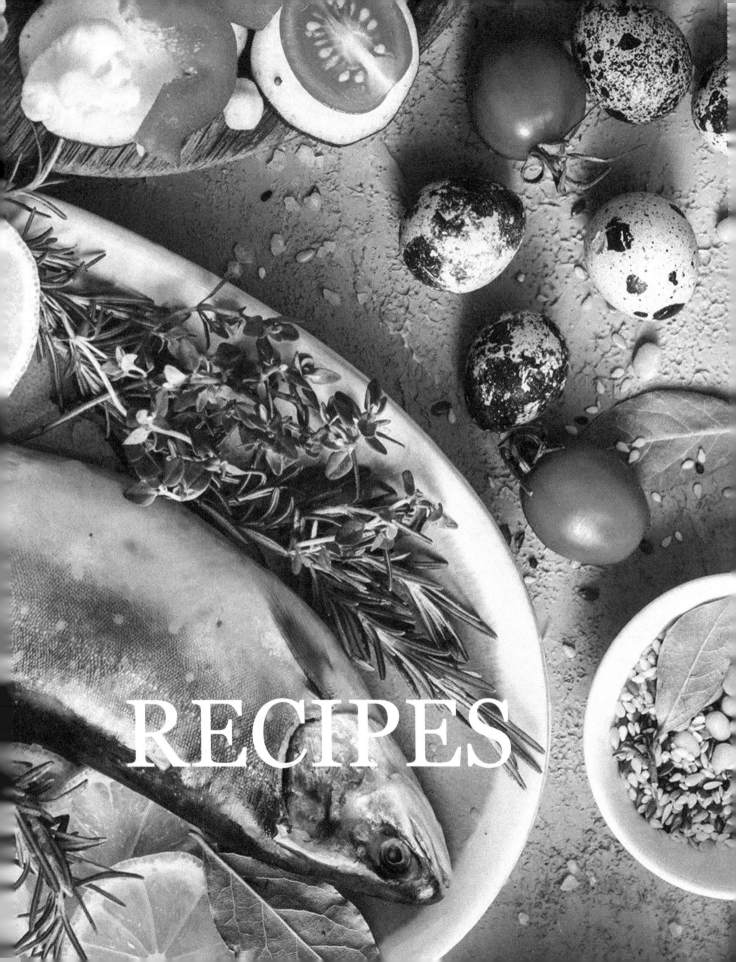

RECIPES

Bread, Pizza & More

Oatmeal Raisin Orange Bread

COOKING: 60+ MIN

SERVES: 6

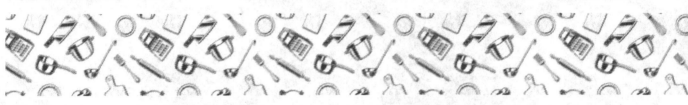

INGREDIENTS

2 cups quick-cooking oats
1/2 cup raisins
2 1/2 cups water, divided
1 (.25 ounce) package active dry yeast
1/2 cup orange juice
1/2 cup molasses
1/3 cup olive oil
1 tablespoon salt
6 cups all-purpose flour
1 egg
1 tablespoon milk

Nutritional Value: 122 calories per serving

DIRECTIONS

1. Place oats and raisins in a bowl. Heat 2 cups water to 120 degrees F-130 degrees F; pour over oats and raisins. Cool to 110 degrees F, about 10 minutes. Place yeast in a small bowl. Heat remaining water to 110 degrees F-115 degrees F; pour over yeast to dissolve. Add to oat mixture. Add the orange juice, molasses, oil, salt and 3 cups flour; beat until smooth. Stir into enough remaining flour to form a soft dough. Turn onto a floured surface; knead until smooth and elastic, about 6-8 minutes. Place in a greased bowl, turning once to grease top. Cover and let rise in a warm place until doubled, about 1-1/2 hours. Punch dough down. Turn onto a lightly floured surface; divide into thirds. Shape each into a round or oval loaf. Place on greased baking sheets. Cover and let rise until doubled, about 45 minutes. With a sharp knife, make three to five shallow slashes across the top of each loaf. Beat egg and milk; lightly brush over loaves. Bake at 350 degrees F for 35-40 minutes or until golden brown. Remove from pans to wire racks to cool.

Bread, Pizza & More

Banana Strawberry Loaf

COOKING: 60+ MIN

SERVES: 10+

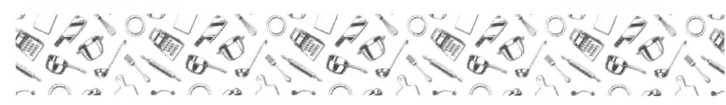

INGREDIENTS

2 cups quick-cooking oats
1/2 cup raisins
2 1/2 cups water, divided
1 (.25 ounce) package active dry yeast
1/2 cup orange juice
1/2 cup molasses
1/3 cup olive oil
1 tablespoon salt
6 cups all-purpose flour
1 egg
1 tablespoon milk

Nutritional Value: 122 calories per serving

DIRECTIONS

1.   Place oats and raisins in a bowl. Heat 2 cups water to 120 degrees F-130 degrees F; pour over oats and raisins. Cool to 110 degrees F, about 10 minutes. Place yeast in a small bowl. Heat remaining water to 110 degrees F-115 degrees F; pour over yeast to dissolve. Add to oat mixture. Add the orange juice, molasses, oil, salt and 3 cups flour; beat until smooth. Stir into enough remaining flour to form a soft dough. Turn onto a floured surface; knead until smooth and elastic, about 6-8 minutes. Place in a greased bowl, turning once to grease top. Cover and let rise in a warm place until doubled, about 1-1/2 hours. Punch dough down. Turn onto a lightly floured surface; divide into thirds. Shape each into a round or oval loaf. Place on greased baking sheets. Cover and let rise until doubled, about 45 minutes. With a sharp knife, make three to five shallow slashes across the top of each loaf. Beat egg and milk; lightly brush over loaves. Bake at 350 degrees F for 35-40 minutes or until golden brown. Remove from pans to wire racks to cool.

Bread, Pizza & More

Oatmeal Raisin Orange Bread

COOKING: 60+ MIN

SERVES: 10+

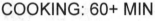
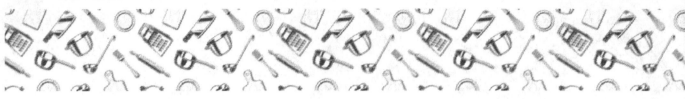

INGREDIENTS

2 cups whole wheat flour
1 teaspoon baking soda
2 eggs
5/8 cup vegetable oil, divided
1 1/2 cups white sugar
3 bananas, mashed
1 cup chopped strawberries
1 pinch ground cinnamon

Nutritional Value: 133 calories per

serving

DIRECTIONS

1. Preheat oven to 350 degrees F (175 degrees C). Lightly grease and flour loaf pan.
2. In a large bowl combine flour, baking soda and cinnamon. Set aside.
3. In a medium bowl blend together with an electric mixer the oil, sugar, eggs and banana until well combined.
4. Add banana mix to the flour mix. Add the strawberries. Mix with a spoon until combined. Do not overmix.
5. Pour the mix into the loaf pan and bake at 350 degrees F (175 degrees C) for 1 hour and 15 minutes or until a toothpick inserted in the center comes out clean and the loaf is well browned. Note: Blueberries or chocolate chips are great in place of the strawberries

Bread, Pizza & More

Strawberry Bread

COOKING: 60+ MIN

SERVES: 4

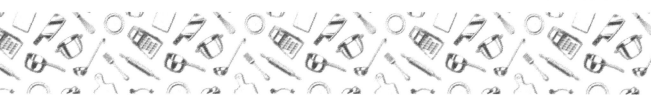

INGREDIENTS

2 cups fresh strawberries
3 1/8 cups all-purpose flour
2 cups white sugar
1 tablespoon ground cinnamon
1 teaspoon salt
1 teaspoon baking soda
1 1/4 cups vegetable oil
4 eggs, beaten
1 1/4 cups chopped pecans

Nutritional Value: 120 calories per serving

1.

DIRECTIONS

1. Preheat oven to 350 degrees F (175 degrees C). Butter and flour two 9 x 5-inch loaf pans.
2. Slice strawberries, and place in medium-sized bowl. Sprinkle lightly with sugar and set aside while preparing bread mixture.
3. Combine flour, sugar, cinnamon, salt and baking soda in large bowl: mix well. Blend oil and eggs into strawberries. Add strawberry mixture to flour mixture, blending until dry Ingredients are just moistened. Stir in pecans. Divide batter into pans.
4. Bake for 45 to 50 minutes, or until tester inserted comes out clean. Let cool in pans on wire rack for 10 minutes. Turn loaves out, and cool completely.

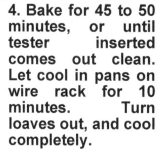

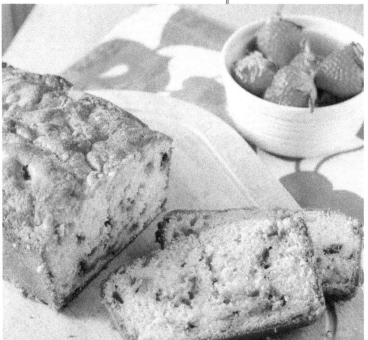

Bread, Pizza & More

Bread with Pears

COOKING: 60+ MIN

SERVES: 10+

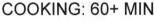

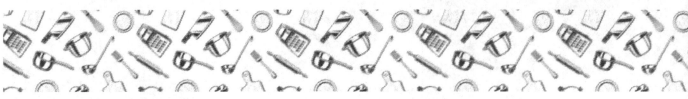

INGREDIENTS

3 1/2 cups all-purpose flour
1 teaspoon baking powder
1 teaspoon salt
1 teaspoon ground ginger
1/2 teaspoon baking soda
1/2 teaspoon ground nutmeg
1 1/2 cups sugar
1/2 cup vegetable oil
1/2 cup butter or margarine, melted
4 eggs
2 teaspoons vanilla extract
2 cups diced peeled pears

Nutritional Value: 100 calories per serving

DIRECTIONS

1. In a large bowl, combine the flour, baking powder, salt, ginger, baking soda and nutmeg; set aside. In a mixing bowl, beat the sugar, oil and butter. Add eggs, one at a time, beating well after each addition. Stir in vanilla. Stir into dry Ingredients just until moistened (batter will be stiff). Stir in pears. Pour into two greased 8-in. x 4-in. x 2-in. loaf pans. Bake at 350 degrees F for 55-65 minutes or until a toothpick comes out clean. Cool for 10 minutes before removing from pans to wire racks..

Bread, Pizza & More

Onion Focaccia

COOKING: 60+ MIN

SERVES: 6+

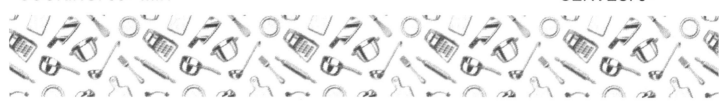

INGREDIENTS

3/4 cup water (70 to 80 degrees F)
2 tablespoons olive oil
1 teaspoon salt
2 cups bread flour 1 tablespoon sugar
1 1/2 teaspoons active dry yeast
2 medium onions, quartered and sliced
3 garlic cloves, minced
1/4 cup butter
2 teaspoons Italian seasoning
1 cup shredded Cheddar cheese
2 tablespoons grated Parmesan cheese

Nutritional Value: 130 calories per serving

DIRECTIONS

1. In bread machine pan, place the first six Ingredients in order suggested by manufacturer. Select dough setting (check dough after 5 minutes of mixing; add 1 to 2 tablespoons of water or flour if needed).
2. When the cycle is completed, turn dough onto a lightly greased 12- in. pizza pan; pat into a 10-in. circle. Cover and let rise in a warm place until doubled, about 30 minutes. Meanwhile, in a large skillet, saute onions and garlic in butter for 18-20 minutes or until golden brown. Stir in the Italian seasoning; cook 1 minute longer.
3. Using the end of a wooden spoon handle, make deep indentations 1 in. apart in dough. Top with onion mixture and cheeses. Bake at 400 degrees F for 15-18 minutes or until golden brown. Serve warm.

Bread, Pizza & More

Nut Bread with Oranges

COOKING: 60+ MIN

SERVES: 10+

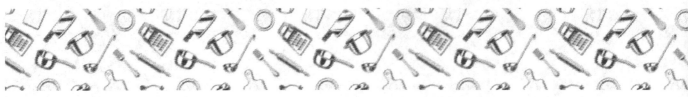

INGREDIENTS

1 tablespoon grated orange zest
1/3 cup fresh orange juice
2/3 cup hot water
2 tablespoons melted shortening
1 teaspoon vanilla extract
1 egg
2 cups all-purpose flour
1/4 teaspoon salt
1 teaspoon baking powder
1/2 teaspoon baking soda
1 cup raw honey
1/2 cup chopped walnuts

Nutritional Value: 145 calories per serving

DIRECTIONS

1. Preheat oven to 350 degrees F (175 degrees C). Grease 3 to 4 mini loaf pans (5x3 inches each).
2. Zest and juice an orange; set 1 tablespoon zest aside. Pour orange juice into a one-cup measuring cup, add boiling water to fill to one cup measurement.
3. Pour juice mixture into a bowl and add the melted shortening, vanilla, egg, flour, salt, baking powder, baking soda, sugar, grated orange zest and chopped nuts. Stir well and pour batter into the prepared pans.
4. Bake at 350 degrees F (175 degrees C) for 45 minutes or until a toothpick comes out clean and bread is nicely browned.

Bread, Pizza & More

The Perfect Italian Bread

COOKING: 60+ MIN

SERVES: 10+

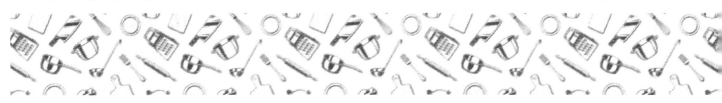

INGREDIENTS

1 tbsp. sugar
2 tsp. salt
2 packages active dry yeast
cornmeal
5 cups all-purpose flour
1 tbsp. butter
water
salad oil
1 egg white

Nutritional Value: 65 calories per

serving

DIRECTIONS

1. In large bowl, combine sugar, salt, yeast and 2 cups flour. In 1-quart saucepan over low heat, heat butter and 1-3/4 cups water until very warm (butter doesn't need to melt).
2. With mixer at low speed, gradually beat liquid into dry
3. Ingredients until just blended. Increase speed to medium, beat 2 minutes.
4. Beat in 1/2 cup flour to make thick batter. Continue beating mixture at medium for 2 minutes. Scrape bowl often with spatula.
5. With wooden spoon, stir in enough additional flour (about 1-3/4 cups) to make a soft dough.
6. Turn dough onto floured surface, knead until smooth and elastic, about 10 minutes, adding flour while kneading.
7. Cut dough in half, cover pieces with bowl. Let dough rest 20 minutes for easier shaping.
8. Grease large cookie sheet; sprinkle with cornmeal.
9. On floured surface with floured rolling pin, roll each half into
10. 15" by 10" rectangle. From 15" side, tightly roll dough, pinch seam to seal.
11. Place loaves, seam side down, on cookie sheet and taper ends.
12. Brush loaves with oil; cover loosely with plastic wrap.
13. Refrigerate 2 - 24 hours.
14. Preheat oven to 425 degrees. Remove loaves from fridge, uncover.
15. Let stand 10 minutes. cut 3 or 4 diagonal slashes on top of each loaf. Bake 20 minutes.
16. In small bowl with fork, beat egg white with 1 tbsp. water.
17. Remove loaves from oven, brush with egg, return to oven, bake 5 minutes.

Bread, Pizza & More

Croissant Bread with Cherries

COOKING: 60+ MIN

SERVES: 10+

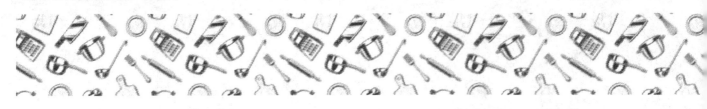

INGREDIENTS

1 tablespoon butter, softened
3 eggs, lightly beaten
1 1/2 cups half-and-half or light cream
1 1/2 teaspoons almond extract
6 medium croissants, halved horizontally
1 cup semisweet chocolate pieces, ground
1 (21 ounce) can Cherry Pie Filling
1 cup sliced almonds Vanilla ice cream (optional)

Nutritional Value: 195 calories per serving

DIRECTIONS

1. Preheat oven to 350 degrees F. Spread butter on bottom and sides of a 9- to 10-inch deep-dish pie plate. In a shallow container Mix eggs, half-and-half, and almond extract; add croissants. Let soak 3 minutes, turning once. Place bottom halves of croissants, slice-side-up, in the prepared dish. Sprinkle with 1/2 of the chocolate. Spoon on 1/2 cup Cherry Pie Filling and 1/2 cup of the nuts. Add croissant tops, slice-sides down, remaining chocolate, another 1/2 cup pie filling and the remaining nuts. Pour on any remaining egg mixture.
2. Bake, uncovered, for 40 to 45 minutes or until center is set. Cool on wire rack about 30 minutes.
3. Heat remaining Cherry Pie Filling and pass with bread pudding. Serve with ice cream, if desired.

Bread, Pizza & More

Orange Bread with Apricots

COOKING: 60+ MIN

SERVES: 10+

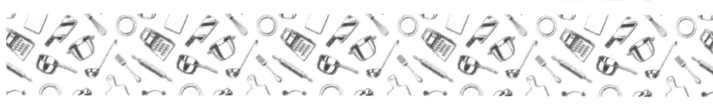

INGREDIENTS

2 cups all-purpose flour
1 tablespoon baking powder
1/2 teaspoon salt
1/4 teaspoon baking soda
3/4 cup raw honey
1/4 cup butter or olive oil, softened
1/2 cup orange juice
2 tablespoons milk
1 egg
1 1/2 cups dried apricots, chopped
1/2 cup semisweet chocolate chips
1/2 cup chopped walnuts

Nutritional Value: 133 calories per serving

DIRECTIONS

1. Preheat oven to 350 degrees F (175 degrees C). Grease a 9x5 inch loaf pan. Sift together flour, baking powder, salt and baking soda, set aside.
2. In a large bowl, cream together the butter or olive oil and sugar until light and fluffy. Add the orange juice, milk and egg; beat well. Gradually blend in the flour mixture. Stir in the apricots, chocolate chips and walnuts. Pour batter into the prepared pan.
3. Bake at 350 degrees F (175 degrees C) for 50 to 55 minutes, or until a toothpick inserted into the center of the loaf comes out clean.
4. Cool loaf in the pan for 10 minutes before removing to a wire rack to cool completely.

Bread, Pizza & More

Almond Herb Bread

COOKING: 60+ MIN

SERVES: 10+

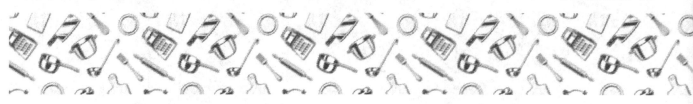

INGREDIENTS

1 (.25 ounce) package active dry yeast
2 tablespoons sugar
1/4 cup warm water (105 degrees to 115 degrees)
1/4 cup butter or margarine
1 teaspoon salt
1 cup warm milk (110 to 115 degrees F)
3 1/2 cups all-purpose flour, divided
1 teaspoon dried rosemary, crushed
1 teaspoon dill weed
1/2 teaspoon dried marjoram, crushed
1/2 cup finely chopped almonds, toasted, divided
1 egg, beaten
1 tablespoon water

Nutritional Value: 136 calories per serving

DIRECTIONS

1. Dissolve yeast and sugar in warm water; set aside. In large mixing bowl, combine butter, salt and milk.
2. Stir in yeast mixture, 2 cups flour, herbs and 2 tablespoons almonds. Beat until well-mixed.
3. Stir in enough remaining flour to form a soft dough. Turn out onto a floured surface and knead until smooth and elastic, about 6-8 minutes. Place dough in greased bowl, turning once to grease dough surface.
4. Cover.
5. Let rise in warm place until doubled, about 1 hour. Punch dough down and cut off 1/3 of dough; set aside.
6. Divide remaining dough into three equal parts, shaping each into a 14-in. rope. Braid ropes and place on greased baking sheet.
7. Divide set- aside dough into three ropes and braid. Place smaller braid on top of larger braid.
8. Cover; let rise until doubled, about 1 hour.
9. Combine egg and water.
10. Brush over entire loaf; sprinkle with remaining almonds. Bake at 375 degrees F for 30 minutes.

Bread, Pizza & More

Sweet Bread with Almonds

COOKING: 60+ MIN

SERVES: 10+

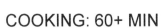

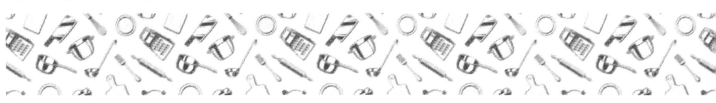

INGREDIENTS

Dough:
2/3 cup warm milk (70 to 80 degrees F)
1 egg yolk
1/4 cup butter or margarine, softened
1/4 cup applesauce, room temperature
1/3 cup sugar
1/2 teaspoon salt
2 3/4 cups bread flour
2 1/4 teaspoons active dry yeast
Topping:
1/4 cup butter
 3 tablespoons sugar
1 tablespoon milk
1/4 teaspoon ground cinnamon
1/8 teaspoon salt
6 tablespoons sliced almonds

Nutritional Value: 133

calories per serving

DIRECTIONS

1. In bread machine pan, place dough Ingredients in order suggested by manufacturer. Select dough setting (check dough after 5 minutes of mixing; add 1 to 2 tablespoons of water or flour if needed). When cycle is completed, turn dough onto a floured surface and punch down. Divide dough in half. Roll each portion into a 6-in. circle and place on greased baking sheets. Cover and let rise in a warm place until doubled, about 30 minutes. Meanwhile, for topping, combine butter, sugar, milk, cinnamon and salt in a small saucepan. Cook and stir over low heat until butter is melted. Simmer for 1 minute.
2. Remove from the heat; cool for 5 minutes. Make a 1/4-in. depression in the center of each loaf with the tip of a wooden spoon. Brush with butter mixture and sprinkle with almonds. Bake at 375 degrees F for 18-20 minutes or until golden brown. Cool for 10 minutes. Serve warm.

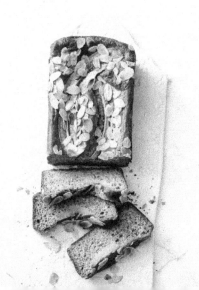

Bread, Pizza & More

Pecan Pear Bread

COOKING: 60+ MIN

SERVES: 10+

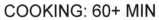

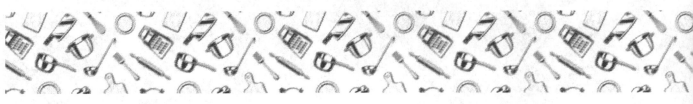

INGREDIENTS

1 cup sugar
1/2 cup vegetable oil
2 eggs
1/4 cup sour cream
1 teaspoon vanilla extract
2 cups all-purpose flour
1 teaspoon baking soda
1/2 teaspoon salt
1/4 teaspoon ground cardamom
1/4 teaspoon ground cinnamon
1 1/2 cups chopped peeled pears
2/3 cup chopped pecans
1/2 teaspoon grated lemon peel

Nutritional Value: 145 calories per serving

DIRECTIONS

1. In a mixing bowl, combine sugar and oil. Add eggs, one at a time, beating well after each addition. Add sour cream and vanilla; mix well. Combine dry Ingredients; add to sour cream mixture and mix well. Stir in pears, pecans and lemon peel.
2. Spread into a greased 8-in. x 4-in. x 2-in. loaf pan. Bake at 350 degrees F for 65-75 minutes or until a toothpick inserted near the center comes out clean. Cool for 10 minutes; remove from pan to a wire rack to cool completely.

Bread, Pizza & More

Cranberry Pecan Bread

COOKING: 60+ MIN

SERVES: 10+

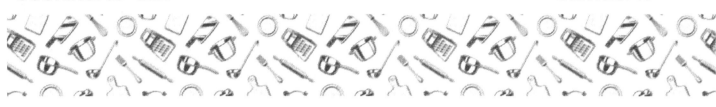

INGREDIENTS

3/4 cup coarsely chopped pecans
3/4 cup dried cranberries
1 1/2 cups all-purpose flour
1 1/2 cups bread flour
1 cup water (75 to 85 degrees F)
3/4 cup sourdough starter*
1 1/2 teaspoons salt
1 tablespoon melted butter

Nutritional Value: 245 calories per

serving

DIRECTIONS

1. Preheat an oven to 275 degrees F (135 degrees C). Spread the pecans onto a baking sheet, and toast until the nuts start to turn golden brown and become fragrant, about 45 minutes. Watch the nuts carefully as they bake, because they burn quickly. Once toasted, set the nuts aside to cool.
2. Cover the cranberries with hot water and allow to soak while you are making the dough.
3. Mix the all-purpose flour and bread flour with the water in the bowl of a stand mixer or a mixing bowl and combine to make a rough dough. Cover the bowl with plastic wrap and allow to rest for 30 minutes.
4. Mix in the sourdough starter and salt, and knead until the dough is smooth and elastic, 3 to 5 minutes if using the stand mixer, or 9 to 11 minutes by hand.
5. Drain the cranberries and knead them into the dough, along with the pecans. Knead another 1 or 2 more minutes, to fully incorporate them into the dough. Lightly oil a large bowl, then place the dough in the bowl and turn to coat with oil. Cover with a light cloth and let rise in a warm place (80 to 95 degrees F (27 to 35 degrees C)) until doubled in volume, 4 to 6 hours.
6. Do not punch down dough. Scrape the risen dough onto a lightly floured work surface, and form into a round loaf. Let rest for 10 minutes. Shape the dough into a round or oblong loaf, place the loaf on a sheet of parchment paper, lightly dust with flour, and let rise until it nearly doubles in size, 1 to 2 more hours.
7. Preheat oven to 400 degrees F (200 degrees C). If using a baking or pizza stone, let it heat in the oven at least 45 minutes before baking.
8. Brush the top of the loaf with water, and make shallow cuts in the loaf with a sharp knife. Place the loaf and parchment paper into the oven, on top of a baking sheet or stone, and bake until brown and the loaf sounds hollow when tapped, 30 to 35 minutes. Remove the loaf to a cooling rack, brush with melted butter, and let cool for at least 1 hour before slicing.

Bread, Pizza & More

Pecan Pumpkin Bread with Chocolate

COOKING: 60+ MIN

SERVES: 10+

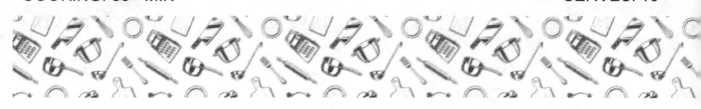

INGREDIENTS

3 cups all-purpose flour
1 teaspoon baking soda
1/2 teaspoon baking powder
1 1/2 teaspoons ground cinnamon
1 teaspoon ground nutmeg
1/2 teaspoon salt
2 cups canned pumpkin
2 1/2 cups white sugar 1 cup
vegetable oil
4 beaten eggs
1 cup chopped pecans
1 cup miniature chocolate chips

Nutritional Value: 166 calories per

serving

DIRECTIONS

1. Preheat oven to 350 degrees F (175 degrees C). Grease two 8x4 inch loaf pans.
2. Sift together the flour, baking soda, baking powder, cinnamon, nutmeg, and salt in a bowl.
3. In another bowl, mash the pumpkin, and stir in the sugar, oil, and eggs. Pour the flour mixture into the pumpkin mixture and stir lightly to combine. Use a rubber spatula to fold the pecans and chocolate chips into the batter. Gently run the spatula through the center of the bowl, then around the sides of the bowl, repeating until fully incorporated.
4. Fill the prepared loaf pans about 3/4 full and bake in the preheated oven for 20 to 25 minutes, until the bread has risen, and a toothpick inserted into the center comes out clean. Cool in the pans for 10 minutes before removing to cool completely on a wire rack.

Bread, Pizza & More

Nut Bread with Strawberries

COOKING: 60+ MIN

SERVES: 10+

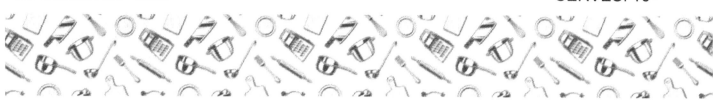

INGREDIENTS

3 cups all-purpose flour
1 teaspoon baking soda
1/2 teaspoon salt
3 teaspoons ground cinnamon
2 cups white sugar
2 cups sliced fresh strawberries
4 eggs
1 1/4 cups vegetable oil
1 cup chopped walnuts

Nutritional Value: 258 calories per serving

DIRECTIONS

1. Preheat oven to 350 degrees F (175 degrees C). Lightly grease 2 9x5 inch loaf pans.
2. Sift together the flour, baking soda, salt, ground cinnamon and sugar in a large mixing bowl. Make a well in the center. Beat together the eggs and oil and pour them into the well. Stir just enough to moisten the Ingredients. Fold in the strawberries and nuts. Pour mixture into prepared pans, fill containers no more than half full.
3. Bake in a preheated oven about 60 minutes or until a toothpick inserted in the center comes out clean. Cool 20 to 30 minutes before removing from pans. Move to a rack to cool completely before slicing.

Bread, Pizza & More

Veggie Pizza

COOKING: 60+ MIN

SERVES: 5+

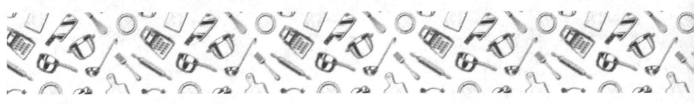

INGREDIENTS

2 (8 ounce) packages refrigerated crescent rolls
1 cup sour cream
1 (8 ounce) package cream cheese, softened
1 teaspoon dried dill weed
1/4 teaspoon garlic salt
1 (1 ounce) package ranch dressing mix
1 small onion, finely chopped
1 stalk celery, thinly sliced
1/2 cup halved and thinly sliced radishes
1 red bell pepper, chopped
1 1/2 cups fresh broccoli, chopped
1 carrot, grated

Nutritional Value: 147 calories per serving

DIRECTIONS

1. Preheat oven to 350 degrees F (175 degrees C). Spray a jellyroll pan with non-stick cooking spray.
2. Pat crescent roll dough into a jellyroll pan. Let stand 5 minutes. Pierce with fork.
3. Bake for 10 minutes, let cool.
4. In a medium-sized mixing bowl, combine sour cream, cream cheese, dill weed, garlic salt and ranch dip mix. Spread this mixture on top of the cooled crust. Arrange the onion, carrot, celery, broccoli, radish, bell pepper and broccoli on top of the creamed mixture. Cover and let chill. Once chilled, cut it into squares and serve.

Bread, Pizza & More

Roasted Tomato Pizza

COOKING: 60+ MIN

SERVES: 5+

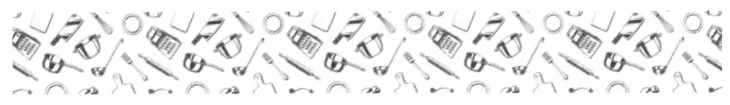

INGREDIENTS

3 cups tom atoes
2 garlic cloves
Fresh thyme leaves
Black Pepper
1 cup parmesan cheese
Sea salt
Whole wheat pita bread

Nutritional Value: 259 calories per

serving

DIRECTIONS

1. Warm up the oven to reach 425° Fahrenheit.
2. Mix the tomatoes, salt, pepper, thyme, garlic, and oil. In a baking pan.
3. Roast for 10 minutes. Pull out the rack from the oven and stir the tomatoes with a wooden spoon or spatula. Mash down to soften the tomatoes and roast for another 10 minutes.
4. Prepare the pita bread with 2 tablespoons of cheese. Arrange them on a large rimmed baking sheet. Toast for the last 5 minutes of the cooking cycle.
5. Remove everything from the oven. Stir the tomatoes and spoon out about one-third of the sauce over each of the pita bread to serve.

Bread, Pizza & More

Greek Pita Pizzas

COOKING: 60+ MIN

SERVES: 5+

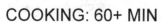

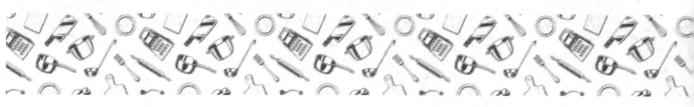

INGREDIENTS

2 tbsp lemon juice
2 pita bread rounds
1.25 cup mozzarella cheese
3 teaspoon olive oil
2 cups fresh spinach
1.25 cup grape tomatoes, halved
6-8 olives, sliced
1.25 teaspoon dried oregano, dried basil, and garlic powder

Nutritional Value: 352 calories per serving

DIRECTIONS

1. Set your oven to 375 degrees F.
2. Mix the herbs, garlic powder, and lemon juice and olive oil into the mixture. Arrange your pita bread and brush with olive oil. You should still have half the mixture left over; you only should use a few drops.
3. In another bowl, Mix the olives, spinach, and tomatoes. Arrange the veggies on the tray and drizzle them with the leftover olive oil Sprinkle your pizza with mozzarella cheese. You can bake anywhere from 6 to 8 minutes until your cheese turns brown.

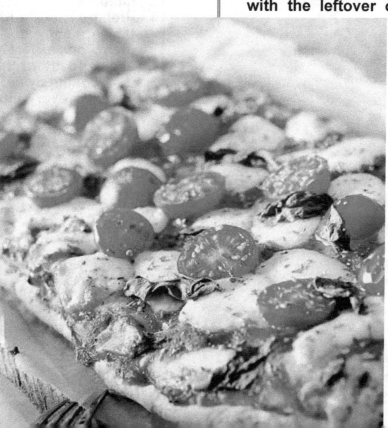

Bread, Pizza & More

Meat Pizzas

COOKING: 60+ MIN

SERVES: 4+

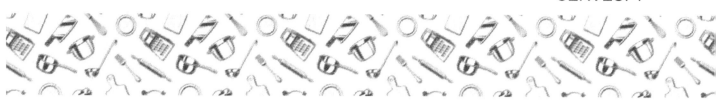

INGREDIENTS

1 stale roll
1/4 cup warm water
2 onions
1 lb. ground beef
1 egg
salt and pepper
1/4 tsp. cayenne pepper
1 - 2 tsp. chili sauce
1/4 cup oil
2 eggs, hard-cooked
2 tomatoes
12 stuffed green olives
4 slices cheese
8 anchovy fillets (opt.)

Nutritional Value: 245 calories per serving

DIRECTIONS

1. Soften roll in warm water, squeeze out water, crumble into small pieces.
2. Peel and finely chop onions, mix with bread, beef, egg, salt, and pepper, cayenne and chili sauce. Divide into 4 portions and form into a patty. Fry patties in oil 3-4 minutes on each side, until crisp. Transfer to baking sheet.
3. Shell and slice eggs. Slice tomatoes and olives. Cut cheese into strips. Top each patty with mixture. Add anchovy fillets (optional) and cheese.
4. Bake at 400 degrees 5 - 7 minutes, until cheese melts.

Bread, Pizza & More

Tomato Spinach Pizza

COOKING: 60+ MIN

SERVES: 5+

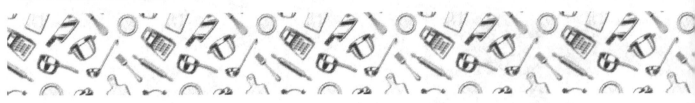

INGREDIENTS

1 1/4 cups water (70 to 80 degrees F)
2 tablespoons olive oil
3/4 teaspoon salt
4 cups all-purpose flour
1 tablespoon active dry yeast
Toppings
1 tablespoon olive oil
3 tablespoons grated Parmesan cheese
1 tablespoon Italian seasoning
3/4 teaspoon garlic salt
1 (10 ounce) package frozen chopped spinach, thawed and squeezed dry
3 plum tomatoes, thinly sliced
2 cups shredded part-skim mozzarella cheese

Nutritional Value: 100 calories per serving

DIRECTIONS

1. In bread machine pan, place the first five Ingredients in order suggested by manufacturer. Select dough setting (check dough after 5 minutes of mixing; add 1 to 2 tablespoons of water or flour if needed).
2. When cycle is completed, turn dough onto a lightly floured surface. Roll into a 16-in. x 11-in. rectangle. Transfer to a 15-in. x 10-in. x 1- in. baking pan coated with nonstick cooking spray. Build up edges slightly. Prick dough thoroughly with a fork. Brush with oil; sprinkle with Parmesan cheese, Italian seasoning and garlic salt. Top with spinach, tomatoes and mozzarella cheese.
3. Bake at 375 degrees F for 17-22 minutes or until crust is golden brown and cheese is melted. Broil 4-6 in. from the heat for 2-3 minutes or until cheese is golden brown.

Bread, Pizza & More

Red, White and Green Pizza

COOKING: 60+ MIN

SERVES: 10+

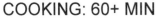

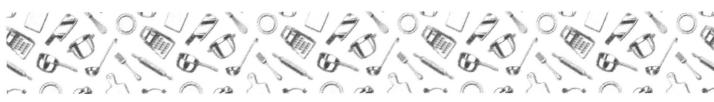

INGREDIENTS

1 (14 ounce) package pizza crust dough
1 teaspoon olive oil
4 ounces ricotta cheese
1/4 cup grated Parmesan cheese
7 ounces frozen chopped spinach, thawed
1 (14 ounce) can artichoke hearts, drained and chopped (optional)
2 cloves garlic, crushed salt and pepper to taste
1 (8 ounce) package shredded Italian 6-cheese blend
2 tomatoes, thinly sliced

Nutritional Value: 324 calories per serving

DIRECTIONS

1. Preheat oven to 375 degrees F (190 degrees C). Lightly grease a baking sheet. Spread the pizza dough in the prepared pan, and rub dough lightly with the olive oil.
2. Stir together the ricotta cheese, Parmesan cheese, spinach, artichoke hearts, garlic, salt, and pepper. Spread the mixture evenly over the dough. Sprinkle evenly with the shredded Italian cheese; top with the sliced tomatoes.
3. Bake in the preheated oven until crust is lightly browned and the cheese is melted and bubbly, about 20 minutes.

Bread, Pizza & More

Mediterranean Pizza

COOKING: 60+ MIN

SERVES: 10+

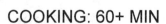

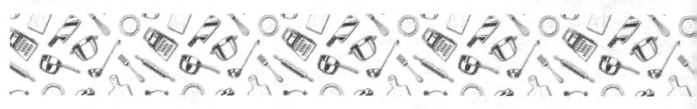

INGREDIENTS

2 (6.5 ounce) jars marinated artichoke hearts
1 (1 pound) loaf frozen bread dough, thawed
1 teaspoon dried basil
1 teaspoon dried oregano
1/2 teaspoon dried thyme
2 cups shredded Monterey Jack cheese, divided
1/4 pound thinly sliced deli ham, julienned
1 cup halved cherry tomatoes
1 cup chopped ripe olives
1/4 cup crumbled feta cheese

Nutritional Value: 471 calories per serving

DIRECTIONS

1. Drain artichokes, reserving marinade. Chop artichokes; set aside. On a floured surface, roll bread dough into a 15-in. circle. Transfer to a greased 14-in. pizza pan; build up edges slightly. Brush up edges slightly. Brush the dough lightly with reserved marinade.
2. Combine the basil, oregano and thyme, sprinkle over marinade. Sprinkle with 1 cup Monterey Jack cheese, ham, artichokes, tomatoes, olives and feta cheese. Sprinkle with remaining Monterey Jack cheese. Bake at 400 degrees F for 20-25 minutes or until crust and cheese are lightly browned.

Bread, Pizza & More

Spinach, Feta and Olives Pizza

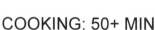

COOKING: 50+ MIN

SERVES: 4+

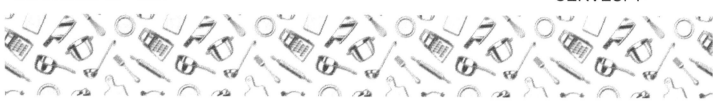

INGREDIENTS

1/2 cup mayonnaise
4 cloves garlic, minced
1 cup crumbled feta cheese, divided
1 (12 inch) pre-baked Italian pizza crust
1/2 cup oil-packed sun-dried tomatoes, coarsely chopped
1 tablespoon oil from the sun- dried tomatoes
1/4 cup pitted kalamata olives, coarsely chopped
1 teaspoon dried oregano
2 cups baby spinach leaves
1/2 small red onion, halved and thinly sliced

Nutritional Value: 236 calories per serving

DIRECTIONS

1. Adjust oven rack to lowest position, and heat oven to 450 degrees. Mix mayonnaise, garlic and 1/2 cup feta in a small bowl. Place pizza crust on a cookie sheet; spread mayonnaise mixture over pizza, then top with tomatoes, olives and oregano. Bake until heated through and crisp, about 10 minutes.
2. Toss spinach and onion with the 1 Tb. sun-dried tomato oil. Top hot pizza with spinach mixture and remaining 1/2 cup feta cheese.
3. Return to oven and bake until cheese melts, about 2 minutes longer. Slice into 6 slices and serve.

Bread, Pizza & More

Baked Potato Pizza

COOKING: 60+ MIN

SERVES: 5+

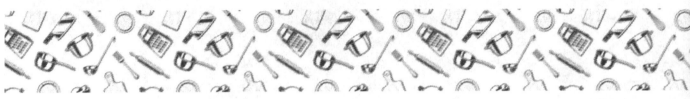

INGREDIENTS

1 (6.5 ounce) package pizza crust mix

3 medium unpeeled potatoes, baked and cooled

1 tablespoon butter or olive oil, melted

1/4 teaspoon garlic powder

1/4 teaspoon dried Italian seasoning

1 cup sour cream

6 bacon strips, cooked and crumbled

3 green onions, chopped

1 1/2 cups shredded mozzarella cheese

1/2 cup shredded Cheddar cheese

Nutritional Value: 147 calories per serving

DIRECTIONS

1. Prepare crust according to package Instructions. Press dough into a lightly greased 14-in. pizza pan; build up edges slightly. Bake at 400 degrees F for 5-6 minutes or until crust is firm and begins to brown.
2. Slice potatoes into 1/2-in. cubes. In a bowl, Mix butter, garlic powder and Italian seasoning. Add potatoes and toss. Spread sour cream over crust, top with potato mixture, bacon, onions and cheeses. Bake at 400 degrees F for 15-20 minutes or until cheese is lightly browned.

Bread, Pizza & More

Black Bean and Spinach Pizza

COOKING: 40+ MIN

SERVES: 5+

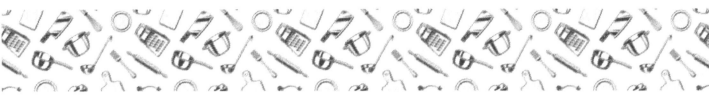

INGREDIENTS

1 (10 ounce) package prebaked Italian bread shell crust
1 (15 ounce) can black beans, rinsed, drained, and mashed
1/3 cup chopped onion
2 teaspoons chili powder
1 teaspoon ground cumin
1/2 teaspoon minced garlic
1/2 cup salsa
1/2 cup frozen chopped spinach, thawed and squeezed dry
2 tablespoons minced fresh cilantro
1/2 teaspoon hot pepper sauce
1/2 cup shredded Monterey Jack cheese
1/2 cup shredded sharp Cheddar cheese

Nutritional Value: 313 calories per serving

DIRECTIONS

1. Place the crust on an ungreased 12-in. pizza pan. Combine the beans, onion, chili powder, cumin and garlic; spread over crust. Layer with salsa, spinach and cilantro. Sprinkle with hot pepper sauce and cheeses. Bake at 450 degrees F for 8-10 minutes or until golden brown.

Bread, Pizza & More

Quick Bread with Orange

COOKING: 60+ MIN

SERVES: 4

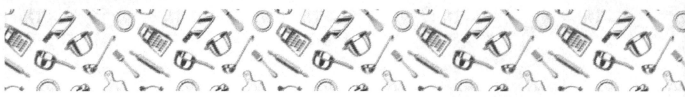

INGREDIENTS

2 cups biscuit baking mix
1/2 cup raw honey
2 tablespoons grated orange zest
2/3 cup orange juice
1 egg, beaten
1 tablespoon olive oil
1/2 cup almonds, chopped
1/2 cup raisins

Nutritional Value: 147 calories per serving

DIRECTIONS

1. Preheat oven to 350 degrees F (175 degrees C). Lightly grease a 9x5 inch loaf pan.
2. In a large bowl, stir together baking mix, sugar and orange zest. Add orange juice, egg and olive oil; stir to Mix. Fold in almonds and raisins. Pour batter into prepared pan.
3. Bake in preheated oven for 35 minutes, until a toothpick inserted into center of loaf comes out clean.

Bread, Pizza & More

Loaf from Potatoes and Onions

COOKING: 60+ MIN

SERVES: 10+

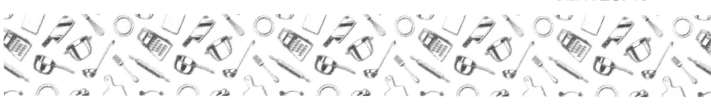

INGREDIENTS

6 baked potatoes
2 eggs, beaten
1 onion, diced
1/2 teaspoon salt
1/2 teaspoon white pepper
1/2 cup shredded sharp Cheddar cheese

Nutritional Value: 240 calories per serving

DIRECTIONS

1. Preheat the oven to 350 degrees F (175 degrees C). Grease an 8x4 inch loaf pan.
2. Remove skins from potatoes, and discard. Place the potatoes in a large bowl, and mash. Mix in onion eggs, salt, pepper and cheese with your hands, or as you would meatloaf. Form into a loaf shape and place into the prepared pan.
3. Bake for 90 minutes in the preheated oven. Let cool for 5 minutes, then remove from the pan, slice and serve.

Bread, Pizza & More

The Mozzarella Bread

COOKING: 60+ MIN

SERVES: 10+

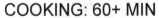

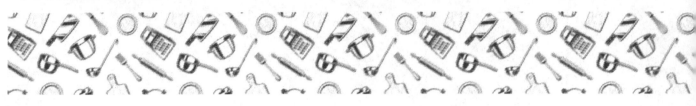

INGREDIENTS

1 long loaf Italian Bread with sesame seed
1 16 oz. package mozzarella cheese
1/2 cup salad olives
1-1/2 tsp. oregano

Nutritional Value: 147 calories per serving

DIRECTIONS

1. Preheat oven to 400 degrees. Cut Italian loaf crosswise into 1"
2. slices. Cut cheese into 1/4" slices. Place cheese and olives between bread slices.
3. Bake bread on cookie sheet for 15 minutes or until cheese is melted. Sprinkle loaf with oregano. Serve immediately.

Bread, Pizza & More

Pecan Oatmeal Loaf

COOKING: 60+ MIN

SERVES: 10+

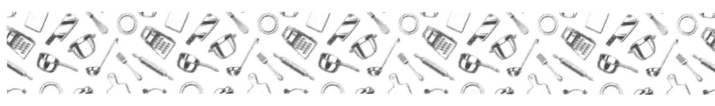

INGREDIENTS

1 1/4 cups water (70 to 80 degrees F)
2 tablespoons butter or margarine,
softened
1/2 cup old-fashioned oats
3 tablespoons sugar
2 tablespoons nonfat dry milk
powder
1 1/4 teaspoons salt
3 cups all-purpose flour
2 teaspoons active dry yeast
1/2 cup chopped pecans

Nutritional Value: 100 calories per
serving

DIRECTIONS

1. In bread machine pan, place the
    first eight Ingredients in order
    suggested by manufacturer. Select
    basic bread setting. Choose crust
    color and loaf size if available. Bake
    according to bread machine
    Instructions (check dough after 5
    minutes of mixing; add 1 to 2
    tablespoons of water or flour if
    needed). Just before the final
    kneading (your machine may
    audibly signal this), add the
    pecans..

Bread, Pizza & More

Bread with Onion and Garlic

COOKING: 60+ MIN

SERVES: 10+

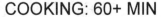

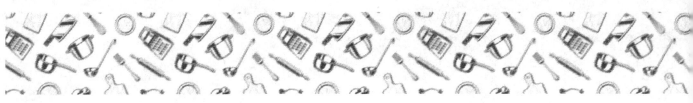

INGREDIENTS

1 (1 pound) loaf frozen bread dough, thawed
1/2 cup finely chopped sweet onion
1/2 cup butter, melted
2 garlic cloves, minced
1 teaspoon dried parsley flakes
1/4 teaspoon salt

Nutritional Value: 145 calories per serving

DIRECTIONS

1. Divide dough into 24 pieces. In a small bowl, combine the remaining Ingredients. Dip each piece of dough into butter mixture; place in a 10-in. fluted tube pan coated with nonstick cooking spray. Cover and let rise in a warm place until doubled, about 1 hour. Bake at 375 degrees F for 20-25 minutes or until golden brown. Serve warm.

Bread, Pizza & More

Onion Garlic Bread

COOKING: 60+ MIN

SERVES: 10+

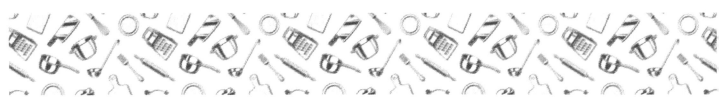

INGREDIENTS

2 French baguettes, cut into 3/4-inch diagonal slices
1 large minced onion
8 cloves minced garlic 1/4 cup butter
2 cups shredded mozzarella cheese
1/2 cup grated Parmesan cheese
1 cup mayonnaise

Nutritional Value: 100 calories per serving

DIRECTIONS

1. Preheat the broiler.
2. Slice the French baguettes diagonally into 3/4-inch slices.
3. In a medium skillet over medium heat, melt the butter. Combine the onions and garlic in the skillet. Cook and stir until tender. Set aside to cool.
4. In a mixing bowl, combine the mozzarella cheese, Parmesan cheese and mayonnaise.
5. On a cookie sheet, arrange the French bread slices in a single layer. Spread the onion and garlic mixture on the bread slices. Spread the cheese and mayonnaise mixture over the onion and garlic mixture on the bread slices. Broil about 5 minutes, until the cheese is bubbly and slightly browned. Serve immediately.

Bread, Pizza & More

Onion Bread with Sauerkraut

COOKING: 60+ MIN

SERVES: 10+

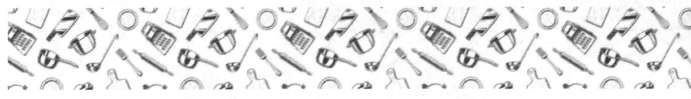

INGREDIENTS

2 1/4 cups bread flour

1 cup milk

3/4 teaspoon salt

1/4 teaspoon onion salt 2 tablespoons
   margarine

1/2 cup sauerkraut - drained, rinsed
   and finely chopped

1 tablespoon finely chopped onion

1/2 cup whole wheat flour

3/4 cup rye flour

1 1/2 tablespoons white sugar

1/2 tablespoon caraway seed

1 3/4 teaspoons active dry yeast

Nutritional Value: 144 calories per

serving

DIRECTIONS

1. Add the Ingredients to the bread pan
   in the order listed. Place the bread
   pan into the machine and close the
   lid. Select the basic setting and
   press start.

Bread, Pizza & More

Pecan Bread with Cherries

COOKING: 60+ MIN

SERVES: 10+

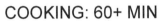
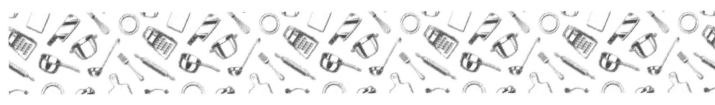

INGREDIENTS

1/2 cup butter or margarine, softened

3/4 cup sugar 2 eggs

2 cups all-purpose flour

1 teaspoon baking soda

1/2 teaspoon salt

1 cup buttermilk

1 cup chopped pecans

1 (10 ounce) jar maraschino cherries, drained and chopped

1 teaspoon vanilla extract

Nutritional Value: 236 calories per serving

DIRECTIONS

1. In a mixing bowl, cream butter and sugar. Add eggs, one at a time, beating well after each addition. Combine the flour, baking soda and salt; add to the creamed mixture alternately with buttermilk. Stir in pecans, cherries and vanilla. Pour into a greased and floured 8-in. x 4-in. x 2-in. loaf pan.

2. Bake at 350 degrees F for 65-75 minutes or until a toothpick inserted near the center comes out clean. Cool for 10 minutes before removing from pan to a wire rack.

Bread, Pizza & More

Poppy Seed Onion Bread

COOKING: 60+ MIN

SERVES: 10+

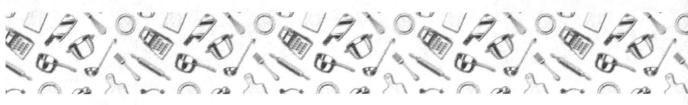

INGREDIENTS

1 1/4 cups water (70 to 80 degrees F)
2 tablespoons butter, softened
2 tablespoons brown sugar
1/4 cup dried minced onion
1 1/2 teaspoons salt
1 teaspoon poppy seeds
1/2 teaspoon onion powder
1/2 teaspoon pepper
3 cups bread flour
2 tablespoons nonfat dry milk powder
3 teaspoons active dry yeast

Nutritional Value: 145 calories per serving

DIRECTIONS

1. In bread machine pan, place all Ingredients in order suggested by manufacturer. Select basic bread setting. Choose crust color and loaf size if available. Bake according to bread machine Instructions (check dough after 5 minutes of mixing; add 1 to 2 tablespoons of water or flour if needed).